I0792305

Real Food for Optimal Pregnancy Health

The Ultimate Guide to Optimal Nutrition, Health, and Wellness During Pregnancy

Barbara J. Winner

Copyright © Barbara J. Winner, 2024.

All rights reserved. No part of this publication may be reproduced, distributed, or transmitted in any form or by any means, including photocopying, recording, or other electronic or mechanical methods, without the prior written permission of the publisher, except in the case of brief quotations embodied in critical reviews and certain other noncommercial uses permitted by copyright law.

TABLE OF CONTENTS

<u>PREGNANCY COMPLICATIONS</u>

<u>CHAPTER 6</u>
<u>EXERCISE WHILE PREGNANT</u>

<u>CHAPTER 7</u>
<u>STRESS AND PREGNANCY</u>

CHAPTER 1

UNDERSTANDING REAL FOOD FOR PREGNANCY

A nutritious, well-balanced, nutrient-dense diet is essential for the health of both pregnant women and their infants. While prenatal nutrition is not a one-size-fits-all strategy, there are a few crucial aspects to remember when eating throughout pregnancy. Defining Real Food Eating "real food" is widely seen as a healthful practice.

However, the notion of "real food" is ambiguous in the field of nutrition. Here are several ways to determine how "real" your diet is. Nutrient-rich foods, also known as nutrient-dense foods, contain a lot of nutrients.

Macronutrients include carbs, proteins, and lipids, while micronutrients include vitamins and minerals. Nutrient-rich foods are those that include a high concentration of vitamins, minerals, fiber, protein, and/or beneficial fatty acids. On the other hand, if a food lacks many of these components, it is considered nutrient-deficient.

Most real foods are nutrient-dense, which helps to replenish your body. Whole foods are foods that are ingested in their natural form. Most whole foods are free of added sugars, processed carbs, artificial colors or flavors, and other manmade components.

Most entire foods are naturally nutrient-dense; examples include fruits, vegetables, nuts, seeds, legumes, dairy, meat, poultry, and seafood. Unprocessed foods, like whole foods, are not manipulated and appear as they do in nature. In current society, many meals are processed to the point where they are barely distinguishable from their original form and do not meet the concept of a true food.

Why Eat Real Foods While Pregnant?
Consuming real, nutrient-dense, whole foods provides your body with the nutrition it requires to produce a healthy baby. Your baby's health will benefit from your

healthy eating habits and nutrient reserves as a mother. Real foods also assist in preventing anemia during pregnancy and lower the risk of pregnancy issues like gestational diabetes, preeclampsia (high blood pressure), and preterm labor. Optimizing your nutrition throughout pregnancy can also aid with postpartum recovery.

A Well-balanced Pregnancy Diet You can use these ideas to create a healthy, balanced pregnancy diet. Well-balanced meals and snacks are essential for a healthy diet in general, but they are especially crucial during pregnancy. In general, including actual foods in nutritious meals and snacks is a good approach to sustaining your body during pregnancy.

Consume nutrient-dense foods, such as fruits and vegetables, to maintain a balanced diet. Complex carbs provide iron, B vitamins, folate, and fiber. Lean proteins promote your baby's optimal growth and development. Healthy fats to meet your energy needs and help your baby's brain develop.

Certain micronutrients are especially crucial during pregnancy. One necessary nutrients are Vitamin A benefits your baby's vision and immune system. Vitamin D helps your baby's bones develop. Calcium works with vitamin D to build your baby's teeth, bones, muscles, heart, and nerves. Choline benefits your baby's brain development. Folate benefits your baby's developing brain and spinal cord. Iron to help with your pregnancy's increased blood supply.

Simple Changes. While knowing what you should eat is important, knowing what foods to avoid is as beneficial. Limiting processed foods is generally beneficial to everyone, but it is especially important for pregnant women who want to improve their diets. Instead of attempting to skip entire food groupings, make tiny changes within each to make your diet more authentically food-based. Fruits and vegetables eaten whole are the most nutrient-dense.

Frozen fruits and veggies also keep their nutrients and are an excellent choice. Unsweetened dried fruit also has important elements. To avoid extra sugars, seek products that are unsweetened or have no added sugar. Fruit snacks, veggie chips, and other processed foods that appear to contain fruits and vegetables but do not should be limited.

There are two types of carbohydrates: whole grains and processed grains. Whole grains include brown rice, oats, quinoa, whole wheat bread and pasta. These grains are less processed and therefore contain more useful elements. Refined grains include white bread, pasta, and rice, which are highly processed and lacking in nutrition.

Try to eat whole grains as often as possible. Proteins that are minimally processed are widely regarded as the healthiest protein sources. Limiting processed meats (bacon and sausage) improves the overall quality of your diet.

Protein-rich foods during pregnancy include lean cuts of beef or pork, chicken, and shellfish. Plant-based proteins like tofu and lentils are also nutritious options. Eggs and dairy products are also good sources of healthful, whole foods during pregnancy.

Consuming whole eggs and whole-milk dairy products improves overall nutritional intake. Eggs are one of the few concentrated sources of choline, which is essential for your baby's brain. Eating the whole egg gives you the most choline.

Consuming full-fat, whole-milk dairy gives your body the fat it requires to absorb vitamins A, D, E, and K. Healthy fats are an important part of your overall energy requirements when pregnant. Specifically, omega-3 fatty acids are required for proper embryonic brain development. Even more specifically, the omega-3 fatty acid docosahexaenoic acid (DHA) is essential for your baby's brain development.

Nuts, seeds, avocado, and fatty seafood are excellent sources of healthful fats while pregnant. Although fish and shellfish are important sources of protein, healthy fats, and iron, there is a risk of consuming mercury-rich seafood while pregnant. Staying Realistic While following these recommendations is desirable, pregnancy may make it difficult to obtain the nutrition your body needs.

Food cravings are typical and might impact your dietary choices during your pregnancy. Food aversions are also frequent, and they may make some of the meals you know are healthfully unsuitable for you at various stages of your pregnancy.

While it is not a food, your prenatal vitamin is an important element of ensuring you are getting the nutrients you require, regardless of what foods are practical for you daily. Prenatal vitamins supply you and your baby with critical nutrients for pregnancy, ensuring that you get them daily.

However, the nutrients in your diet have a synergistic impact, and getting your nutrients from food is generally preferable to taking food supplements. Continue to take your prenatal vitamins, but also make an effort to consume a range of whole foods. If you need help determining which prenatal vitamins to take, consult your doctor or a dietician.

CHAPTER 2

NUTRITION WHILE PREGNANT

Diet and Caloric Recommendations To ensure a healthy pregnancy, roughly 300 additional calories are required every day. These calories should come from a well-balanced diet that includes protein, fruits, vegetables, and whole grains. Sugar and fat should be kept to a minimum.

A healthy, well-balanced diet can also assist in alleviating certain pregnancy symptoms, such as nausea and constipation. Fluid Intake During Pregnancy Fluid consumption is a key aspect of pregnancy nutrition.

Follow these guidelines for fluid intake while pregnant: You can get enough fluids by drinking many glasses of water every day, in addition to juices and soups. Speak with your doctor or midwife about limiting your intake of coffee and artificial sweeteners.
Avoid all types of alcohol.

Ideal foods to eat during pregnancy
The foods listed below are good for your health and fetal development during pregnancy:
vegetables: carrots, sweet potatoes, pumpkin, spinach, cooked greens, tomatoes, and red sweet peppers (for vitamin A and potassium).

Fruit: cantaloupe, honeydew, mangoes, prunes, bananas, apricots, oranges, and red or pink grapefruit (for potassium).

Dairy: fat-free or low-fat yogurt, skim or 1% milk, and soymilk (for calcium, potassium, vitamins A and D).

Grains: ready-to-eat cereals or cooked cereals (for iron and folic acid) Proteins include beans and peas, nuts and seeds, lean beef, lamb, and pig, salmon, trout, herring, sardines, and pollock.

Foods to Avoid While Pregnant
Avoid the following foods when pregnant: Unpasteurized milk and its products (soft cheeses such as feta, queso blanco, and fresco, Camembert, brie, or blue-veined cheeses—unless labeled "made with pasteurized milk") Hot dogs and luncheon meats (unless they are heated to boiling before serving).

Raw or undercooked seafood, eggs, and meat. Do not consume sushi made with raw fish. Refrigerated pâtés and meat spreads.

Refrigerated Smoked Seafood

Guidelines For Safe Food Handling When handling and cooking food, adhere to the following general food safety guidelines:
Wash. Before eating, chopping, or cooking with raw vegetables, thoroughly rinse it under running tap water.

Clean. Wash your hands, knives, countertops, and cutting boards after handling and preparing raw foods.

Cook. Cook beef, pig, or poultry to a safe internal temperature as determined by a food thermometer.

Chill. Refrigerate all perishable foods immediately. Prenatal Vitamins and Mineral Supplements Most healthcare doctors or midwives will recommend a prenatal vitamin before or shortly after conception to ensure that all of your nutritional requirements are met. However, a prenatal supplement cannot replace a balanced diet.

The Importance of Folic Acid

The US Public Health Service recommends that all women of reproductive age take 400 micrograms (0.4 mg) of folic acid daily. Folic acid is a vitamin found in certain green leafy vegetables. Many berries, nuts, legumes, citrus fruits, fortified morning cereals Several vitamin supplements. Folic acid can help lower the chance of neural tube abnormalities, which are birth disorders affecting the brain and spine.

Neural tube abnormalities can cause varied degrees of paralysis, incontinence, and even intellectual incapacity. Folic acid is most effective during the first 28 days following conception, when the majority of neural tube abnormalities develop. Unfortunately, you may not be aware that you are pregnant before 28 days. Folic acid intake should begin before conception and continue throughout the pregnancy. Your healthcare professional or midwife will advise you on the optimum amount of folic acid for your specific needs. Women who take anti-epileptic medicines, for example, may require higher folic acid dosages to prevent neural tube abnormalities. They should consult with their doctor before attempting to conceive.

CHAPTER 3

FOODS TO EAT WHILE PREGNANT

For A Healthy Baby Pregnant women must take special care with their food to meet the unborn baby's nutritional needs. Pregnancy is one of the happiest times in a woman's life, yet it may also cause mental and physical stress.

Maintaining a healthy and balanced diet throughout pregnancy is essential for both the mother's and the baby's health! During this time, your body requires additional nutrients to support your baby's wellness.

During the second and third trimesters, you should increase your daily calorie intake by 400-500.

Poor food habits can lead to obesity and an increased risk of birth problems. Pregnant women must be especially careful about what they consume during their pregnancy to meet the baby's particular nutritional needs.

Eating good, nutrient-dense foods can help you and your fetus stay healthy. It also helps you lose weight quickly after giving delivery. So, just for you, I've produced a list of 10 foods you can eat while pregnant!

1. Dairy Products During pregnancy, dairy products are essential. It helps you meet your fetus's additional protein and calcium requirements. Drink at least one glass of milk every day and eat extra Greek yogurt, paneer, and ghee to keep your infant healthy.

2. Eggs Many people believe eggs to be superfoods because of their high vitamin, protein, and mineral content. The proteins found in eggs are beneficial to the developing baby because they produce and repair fetal cells. Additionally, eggs have a high concentration of choline, which is required for the development of the unborn baby's brain and neurological system.

3. Bananas Bananas are rich in folic acid, calcium, potassium, and vitamin B6. They are also high in antioxidants, which can enhance energy levels. As a result, they might be a beneficial addition to your pregnant diet.

4. Sweet potatoes. Sweet potatoes contain a high concentration of beta-carotene, which is turned into vitamin A by the body and is required for cell and tissue growth. Vitamin A also helps to enhance immunity and improve vision. So, eating extra sweet potatoes can be healthy for both the mother and the unborn child.

5. Legumes Legumes are a food group that includes lentils, soybeans, peas, beans, chickpeas, and peanuts. They are a great source of plant-based fiber, protein, folate, calcium, and iron, all of which are essential for pregnant women. Having adequate folate will ensure that your baby is born healthy and protects him or her from future ailments and infections.

6. Nuts Nuts are delicious and high in healthy fats, making them an excellent choice for snacking during pregnancy. They contain brain-boosting omega-3 fatty acids, proteins, fiber, and other critical nutrients that are required for the baby's growth.

7. Orange Juice Orange juice contains folate, potassium, and vitamin C. It can offer your kid essential nutrients, hence preventing a variety of birth abnormalities. The vitamin C in orange juice improves your baby's ability to absorb iron in the body. So, drink one glass of orange juice every day as part of your breakfast.

8. Leafy veggies. Leafy vegetables are nutrient-dense, and we all know that they can help protect the body from a variety of ailments. Green vegetables are an excellent addition to your pregnancy diet due to their high levels of antioxidants, calcium, protein, fiber, folate, vitamins, and potassium.

9. Oatmeal Oatmeal provides a variety of health benefits. Carbohydrates are essential for all of us, particularly pregnant women because they provide quick energy to do daily tasks. Oatmeal contains carbohydrates, selenium, vitamin B, phosphorus, and calcium. So eat it for breakfast during the pregnancy period.

10. Salmon Salmon contains high levels of omega-3 fatty acids, which are beneficial to heart health. A diet rich in omega-3 fatty acids is vital for pregnant women since it aids in the development of the fetus's brain and eyes. Salmon is also high in vitamin D, which is beneficial to both bone health and immunity.

CHAPTER 4

FOODS TO AVOID WHILE PREGNANT

To avoid endangering your kid, be mindful of what you eat. As an expectant woman, you would be advised to incorporate specific items into your diet that are good for you. To help you stay safe, we've compiled a list of items to avoid while pregnant.

Pregnancy causes several physical changes that have a wide range of effects on the baby's growth. When it comes to diet, pregnant women must ensure that they receive enough nutrients to support the baby's healthy development while remaining nourished.

Certain foods that you may have eaten before pregnancy can become dangerous to consume during pregnancy for a variety of reasons. You may be wondering what not to consume when pregnant. As a result, this section will guide you through the various foods you should avoid during pregnancy, as well as the reasons for doing so and safe substitutes.

Foods To Avoid While Pregnant
Avoiding certain foods keeps you and your kid safe and healthy. We've compiled a list of foods to avoid during the first month of pregnancy as well as other months.

1. Mercury-Containing Fish: Sharks, swordfish, king mackerel, and tilefish should be avoided due to high levels of mercury. "Pregnant women should avoid fish that contain mercury, raw meat like sushi, and organ meat." Mercury, an element found in oceans, streams, and lakes, is converted to methylmercury in the human body. It is a neurotoxin that is associated with brain damage and developmental delays in infants. Low-mercury fish options include salmon, catfish, cod, and canned light tuna. According to the US FDA, you can have up to eight to twelve ounces of fish each week, which equals two to three servings. Limit your

consumption of white tuna (albacore) to six ounces per week.

Solution: Choose fish high in omega-3 fatty acids and low in mercury since the high protein, low saturated fats, and many critical nutrients help the child's heart and brain develop and grow properly. You should, however, consult with a doctor or a certified dietician to learn about which fish you can consume.

2. Avoid smoked and refrigerated seafood, such as lox, jerky, nova style, and kippered, as they contain Listeria monocytogenes bacteria. This bacteria causes listeriosis (symptoms include diarrhea and vomiting), which can result in neonatal sickness and even miscarriage or stillbirth. According to the Centers for Disease Control and Prevention (CDC), pregnant women are 10 times more likely to get listeria infection than other people. Furthermore, processed seafood includes significant levels of sodium, which can contribute to elevated blood pressure and swelling of the body parts.

Solution: Use canned smoked seafood on occasion or when fresh fish is unavailable. However, avoid such foods as much as possible.

3. Fish Exposure to Industrial Pollutants: Fish from local streams, lakes, and rivers contain high levels of

polychlorinated biphenyls. Exposure to these toxins may hurt fetal health, resulting in low birth weight, decreased head size, learning impairments, and memory problems. Avoid eating locally caught striped bass, pike, bluefish, salmon, trout, and walleye.

Solution: You can choose freshwater fish. When fishing in a local stream, lake, or river, keep these recommendations in mind. First, verify the cautions for that body of water. You can find this information on the fishing regulations websites or at your local health department. This information applies to fish taken in local waters rather than those accessible in local grocery stores. Avoid uncooked fish since it increases the risk of contracting foodborne infections.

4. Avoid eating raw shellfish, including oysters, clams, and mussels, to prevent seafood-borne diseases and food poisoning. They contain hazardous germs, viruses, and poisons that can make you sick.

Solution: Instead, you can eat cooked shellfish, ensuring that their shells are open.

5. Raw or undercooked eggs: Raw, undercooked, or soft-boiled eggs should be avoided because they contain pathogenic salmonella bacteria that can cause food poisoning. You may get diarrhea, severe vomiting,

headaches, abdominal pain, and a high fever. All of these symptoms are unlikely to damage your baby, but they will weaken your immune system, which may affect the baby's growth. The following items include raw eggs and must be avoided: homemade Caesar dressings, custards, ice creams, mayonnaise and Hollandaise sauces, Béarnaise sauce, Aioli sauce, and sweets such as mousse, tiramisu, and meringue.

Solution: Purchase pasteurized egg products. You can select professionally prepared ice cream, mousse, eggnog, and condiments. Eat fried eggs with firm yolks, a well-cooked omelet, and salads.

6. Raw Meat and Poultry: Uncooked or bloodied meat and poultry can carry Toxoplasma parasite and Salmonella germs, posing a concern. Salmonella raises the likelihood of food poisoning. Toxoplasma causes toxoplasmosis, which presents with flu-like symptoms a few weeks after consuming the meal. It can result in miscarriage or fetal death during birth.

Solution: Make sure your meat and poultry are properly cooked and heated. Eat home-cooked versions, which should be around 160°F for ground meats, 145°F for whole cuts, and 165°F for chicken breasts.

7. Avoid deli foods (also known as ready-to-eat meats) such as sandwich meat, cold cuts, lunch meat, hotdogs, and sliced meats. They are known to contain listeria germs, which can easily pass from the mother to the placenta, causing catastrophic consequences such as fetal death.

Solution: Listeria is killed by pasteurization and high-temperature cooking. Thus, eat deli meats only after reheating them until they are boiling.

8. Consumption of unpasteurized or raw milk during pregnancy is harmful. It has little nutritional value, and raw milk and its products are responsible for a greater proportion of food-borne illnesses. They include deadly bacteria including salmonella, listeria, E.coli, and cryptosporidium, which can be detrimental to you and your baby.

Solution: Purchase only pasteurized milk and its products. Pasteurization involves heating milk at a high temperature, which kills disease-causing microorganisms. If you buy milk from a local vendor, make sure to thoroughly boil it, as high temperatures kill microorganisms. Non-dairy milk alternatives, such as soy milk, rice milk, almond milk, and oat milk, are safer and have equivalent nutritional value.

9. Camembert, Roquefort, Gorgonzola, brie, feta, blue cheese, queso fresco, queso blanco, and panela should be pasteurized before consumption. Listeria can be found in unpasteurized soft cheeses.

Solution: Eat hard cheeses (Cheddar or Swiss cheeses), which do not contain water like soft cheeses. As a result, these cheeses are unlikely to contain bacteria. Pasteurized non-imported soft cheeses are safe for consumption. Pasteurized or unpasteurized soft or blue cheese heated to a steaming temperature can be ingested during pregnancy.

10. Unwashed Fruits and Vegetables: Unwashed fruits and vegetables contain Toxoplasma parasites, which are harmful to developing babies. Toxoplasmosis contaminates the soil where fruits and vegetables are cultivated, and if you eat them raw, you may consume deadly bacteria.

Solution: Thoroughly rinse the fruits and vegetables with running water. Peel away or scrape the surfaces, then cut off any bruised regions that may harbor bacteria. Cook veggies, especially green ones.

11. Raw Sprouts Clover, alfalfa, mung bean, radish, broccoli, sunflower, onion, soybean, and snow pea sprouts should not be consumed fresh. They are

extremely susceptible to listeria, salmonella, and E.coli germs. As you are aware, listeriosis can result in premature birth, miscarriage, stillbirth, and illnesses in neonates. Salmonella and E. coli can cause severe disease.

Solution: Eat sprouts that have been cooked.

12. Non-pasteurized juices: Fruit and vegetable juices that have not been pasteurized, especially those sold in packages, may contain hazardous microorganisms. Not only that, but a glass of freshly squeezed juice may offer a risk if the fruits and vegetables are not well-cleansed.

Solution: Buy pasteurized juices or prepare your own. Wash the fruits and vegetables thoroughly under running water, scrape away dirt with a brush, and remove any bruised parts.

13. Excess Caffeine: Caffeine consumption may raise your risk of miscarriage and low-birth weight kids. You should limit your daily intake to 200mg. Caffeine can also be found in tea, chocolate, and many energy beverages. According to some research findings, caffeine is linked to premature birth and withdrawal symptoms in babies. Soft drinks, diet soda, alcohol, and iced tea should also be avoided during pregnancy.

Solution: Drink decaffeinated beverages, especially during the first trimester, when the risk of miscarriage is highest.

CHAPTER 5

PREGNANCY COMPLICATIONS

A pregnancy complication is defined as any disease or ailment that impairs a person's pregnancy. The greatest thing you can do throughout pregnancy is to seek regular prenatal care, attend all appointments and testing, and communicate your symptoms to your provider. Most pregnancy problems can be avoided if detected early and treated promptly.

What constitutes a pregnancy complication?
Pregnancy complications are medical disorders that might harm your or the fetus's health while pregnant. During pregnancy, your doctor keeps an eye out for any issues. Attending all of your prenatal appointments will help them spot any concerns. Early detection and timely treatment can significantly lessen the likelihood of major consequences.

What causes problems in pregnancy?
Complications during pregnancy might arise for a variety of causes. Preexisting medical issues, as well as new ones produced by pregnancy, might lead to pregnancy difficulties.

What are the most common pregnancy complications? Some common difficulties in early pregnancy include: Ectopic pregnancy is a situation in which the fertilized egg implants outside the uterus (typically in the fallopian tube). The egg cannot develop outside of your uterus, so you will require surgery or medicines to remove the ectopic tissue. Miscarriage is the loss of a pregnancy within the first 20 weeks. About 10% to 20% of pregnancies result in miscarriage. More than 80% of miscarriages occur in the first trimester.

Hyperemesis gravidarum (HG) refers to severe and persistent vomiting during pregnancy. It might cause dehydration and excessive weight loss.

Congenital disorders: If your healthcare professional suspects that the fetus has a health problem or a congenital condition, you are more likely to experience issues during pregnancy. This could signify you need more monitoring or your kid requires special care at birth.

Some of the most prevalent issues in the latter half of pregnancy include: Preeclampsia is a blood pressure condition that occurs in the second part of pregnancy or up to six weeks following delivery. Approximately 10% of people will acquire this while pregnant. It is more likely in persons who have high blood pressure before becoming pregnant. After your kid is born, the complications will begin to subside. Gestational diabetes develops when pregnancy hormones interfere with your metabolism's ability to maintain stable blood sugar levels. During your pregnancy, you will get a glucose screening to detect diabetes.

Most people can manage their blood sugar levels by food and exercise, but some require medication. Typically, the issue resolves after your baby is delivered. Preterm labor occurs before 37 weeks of pregnancy. This can result in your baby being born underweight or with undeveloped organs.

Diseases: A variety of viral and bacterial diseases can cause pregnancy complications. These include UTIs, yeast infections, group B streptococcus, and bacterial vaginosis. Sexually transmitted infections (STIs) can potentially result in pregnancy problems. Certain illnesses can be transmitted to the fetus during pregnancy (TORCH infections).

Vaginal hemorrhage: Heavy or profuse bleeding during pregnancy necessitates quick treatment. If you observe any bleeding during your pregnancy, contact your provider. Placenta previa or placenta accreta: Placental issues can cause problems during pregnancy, labor, and delivery. Low amniotic fluid (oligohydramnios): The fetus is surrounded by less amniotic fluid than is normal for its age. This raises your chances of having a baby too soon. It is more prevalent than polyhydramnios (excess amniotic fluid), which can also result in difficulties.

Depression and anxiety: Severe sadness or stress during pregnancy (or postpartum, after the baby is born) might impair fetal development. If you have any thoughts of causing injury to the fetus or yourself, contact your clinician immediately. Anemia occurs when you do not have enough red blood cells to transport oxygen throughout your body. It causes you to feel fatigued and weak. It is frequent during pregnancy because more red blood cells are required to provide oxygen to the fetus. Iron deficiency is a prevalent cause of anemia.

You can avoid iron shortage by taking supplements or eating more iron-rich foods. These are just a few of the more prevalent pregnancy issues; there are many more. Talk to your prenatal care provider about how you're feeling during your appointments. Having open chats about your symptoms allows them to discover any concerns. If you have a pregnancy issue, your provider may refer you to a maternal-fetal medicine specialist.

Who is at risk of developing pregnancy complications? Anyone can develop complications during their pregnancy. You are at a higher risk if you have a persistent medical condition or sickness before pregnancy.

Examples of health issues or disorders that can create complications during pregnancy include:
- Diabetes.
- Cancer.
- High blood pressure.

Some people have high blood pressure (hypertension) before becoming pregnant, whereas others develop it during the pregnancy. High blood pressure during pregnancy can prevent the placenta from receiving adequate blood. Sexually transmitted infections (STIs). Kidney issues. Epilepsy. Anemia.

Many drugs used to treat chronic health disorders are safe to use during pregnancy. Some drugs may require more frequent monitoring during pregnancy, as well as dosage adjustments. Please consult with your healthcare professional before discontinuing or changing any of your current drugs.

Other variables that may raise your risk of problems during pregnancy include:
- Being older than 35.
- Being younger than the age of twenty.
- Smoking cigarettes and consuming alcoholic beverages.
- Being pregnant with twins, triplets, or multiples.
- Having a history of miscarriage.
- Being obese.
- Being anorexic.
-

Can uterine fibroids lead to pregnancy complications? Uterine fibroids rarely cause difficulties during pregnancy. They can, however, induce early labor or place the fetus in a breech position. If a fibroid prevents your baby from exiting your vagina during delivery, a C-section may be a safer option.

Can birth control pills lead to pregnancy complications? There is no good evidence that taking birth control tablets during early pregnancy is harmful to the fetus. However, you should discontinue any hormonal contraception as soon as you discover you're pregnant. If you suspect you are pregnant, get a pregnancy test immediately.

Medical researchers do not generally evaluate pregnant mothers or fetuses, which is why data on this topic is sparse. Testing how a pregnant individual reacts to using hormonal birth control throughout the pregnancy endangers the fetus.

How do I avoid pregnancy complications?
While some pregnancy issues are beyond your control, you can take steps to reduce your risk of developing them. This includes: Being in good health before pregnancy. This could include better preexisting condition management, achieving a healthier weight, quitting smoking, and other measures. Attend all of your prenatal checkups, ultrasounds, and testing.

Report any concerning or odd symptoms to your pregnancy care provider. Maintaining a healthy lifestyle during pregnancy includes eating nutritious foods, exercising regularly, and abstaining from alcohol and smoking. Trying to reduce stress and get enough rest while pregnant. Taking prenatal vitamins. Do not take any medications unless your pregnancy care provider gives you the okay.

What percentage of pregnancies involve complications? Most people do not have pregnancy issues. According to studies, approximately 8% of pregnancies contain problems that, if left untreated, could endanger you or the fetus. What is the most prevalent complication of teen pregnancy? Certain conditions are more common in people who become pregnant before the age of 15. This includes Premature birth. Anemia. Pregnancy-induced hypertension (PIH) and toxemia.

Cephalopelvic disproportion (your baby's head is larger than the opening in your pelvis). According to research, infant mortality (death) is higher among teenage parents. How many people die from pregnancy-related complications? Every year in the United States, over 700 people die as a result of pregnancy problems. Many of these deaths are deemed preventable if complications are identified and treated promptly.

Heart and cardiovascular disorders, such as high blood pressure, are the leading causes of pregnancy-related deaths. Infection or Sepsis. Excessive bleeding. Pulmonary embolism (PE). According to studies, a rising number of pregnant people in the United States have a chronic health condition before pregnancy, such as hypertension or diabetes. These illnesses increase your risk of difficulties during pregnancy and the first year after. If you have a chronic health condition and are thinking about getting pregnant, please arrange a pre-pregnancy appointment to find out what precautions you should take before conception.

When should I call my doctor?

It is critical to discuss all of your symptoms with your doctor throughout pregnancy. This is the only approach to identify and address potential problems. If you are experiencing heavy bleeding or vaginal fluid leakage, contact your pregnancy care provider immediately.

- If you have a constant, severe headache.
- Experience rapid or severe swelling.
- Experience dizziness or blurred vision.
- You're experiencing abdominal aches and cramps.
- Have a fever, chills, or vomit.
- Feel the fetus moving less than usual.

Hearing you have a pregnancy problem might be frightening. It is reasonable to be concerned about the health of both the fetus and yourself.

The majority of pregnancy issues may be treated, especially if they are detected early. The best thing you can do is attend all of your prenatal checkups, ultrasounds, and testing. Don't be afraid to ask your physician questions concerning your diagnosis; they can help you feel more at peace. Share your symptoms with them so that you can receive the appropriate care as soon as possible.

CHAPTER 6

EXERCISE WHILE PREGNANT

Is it safe to work when pregnant?
Consult your healthcare provider about exercising during pregnancy. Most pregnant women find that exercise is both safe and healthy for themselves and their babies.

If you and your pregnancy are healthy, exercise will not raise your chances of suffering a miscarriage (when a baby dies in the womb before 20 weeks of pregnancy), a premature baby (born before 37 weeks of pregnancy), or a baby born with a low birth weight (less than 5 pounds 8 ounces).

How much exercise do you need while pregnant?
Healthy pregnant women should engage in at least 2½ hours of moderate-intensity aerobic activity per week. Aerobic activities cause you to breathe more deeply and quickly, as well as your heart rate to increase. Moderate intensity indicates that you are active enough to sweat and raise your heart rate.

A fast stroll is a type of moderate-intensity aerobic activity. If you can't converse normally throughout an activity, you're probably working too hard. You don't need to complete all 2½ hours at once. Instead, divide it up throughout the week. For example, exercise for 30 minutes on most or all days. If this seems like a lot, divide the 30 minutes by doing something physical for 10 minutes three times per day.

Why is regular physical activity beneficial during pregnancy?
- Regular exercise can help healthy pregnant women: Maintain their mental and physical wellbeing.
- Physical activity might make you feel better and offer you more energy.
- It also strengthens your heart, lungs, and blood vessels, which helps you stay fit.
- Help you gain the proper amount of weight during pregnancy.

- Relieve some typical pregnant discomforts, such as constipation, back pain, and swelling in your legs, ankles, and feet.
- Help you cope with stress and sleep better. Stress is concern, strain, or pressure that you experience in response to events in your life.
- Help to lower your risk of pregnancy issues such as gestational diabetes and preeclampsia.

Gestational diabetes is a kind of diabetes that can develop when pregnant. It occurs when your body has an excess of sugar (known as glucose) in its blood. Preeclampsia is a form of high blood pressure that some women get after the 20th week of pregnancy or after childbirth. These disorders can raise your chances of having difficulties during pregnancy, such as premature birth (born before 37 weeks).

Help lower your chances of having a cesarean birth (commonly known as c-section). Cesarean birth is a surgical procedure in which your baby is delivered through a cut made by your doctor in your abdomen and uterus. Prepare your body for labor and childbirth.

Prenatal yoga and Pilates can help you practice breathing, meditation, and other relaxation techniques that can help you manage labor discomfort. Regular exercise will help you gain energy and strength to get through labor.

What activities are safe during pregnancy?
If you were healthy and exercised before becoming pregnant, it is usually okay to continue your activities while pregnant. Check with your provider to make sure. For example, if you are a runner, or tennis player, or engage in other forms of strenuous activity, you may be able to continue your activities while pregnant.

As your belly grows later in pregnancy, you may need to adjust your activities or scale back on your workouts. If your provider says you can exercise, choose activities that you enjoy. If you didn't exercise before becoming pregnant, now is an excellent time to begin. Ask your provider about safe activities. Start slowly and gradually increase your fitness level. For example, start with 5 minutes of action per day and gradually increase to 30 minutes per day.

Typically, these activities are safe to do throughout pregnancy:

Walking. A fast walk is an excellent workout that is easy on your joints and muscles. If you're new to exercise, this is an excellent activity.

Swimming and water workouts. The water supports your increasing baby's weight, and moving against it increases your heart rate. It's also gentle on the joints and muscles. If you experience low back pain when doing other activities, consider swimming.

Riding a stationary bicycle. This is safer than riding a standard bicycle when pregnant. Even as your belly develops, a stationary bike is less likely to cause you to fall off.

Yoga and Pilates classes. Tell your yoga or Pilates instructor that you are pregnant. The instructor can assist you in modifying or avoiding positions that are potentially dangerous for pregnant women, such as laying on your stomach or flat on your back (after the first trimester).

Some gyms and community centers provide prenatal yoga and Pilates programs exclusively for pregnant mothers.

Low-impact aerobics classes. During low-impact aerobics, you always keep one foot on the ground or equipment. Low-impact aerobics include strolling, stationary biking, and utilizing an elliptical machine.

Low-impact aerobics put less strain on your body than high-impact aerobics. During high-impact aerobics, both feet leave the ground simultaneously. Running, jumping rope, and jumping jacks are all examples of physical activities. Tell your teacher you're pregnant so they can assist you alter your workout as needed.

Strength training. Strength exercise can help you gain muscle and strengthen your bones. It is okay to exercise with weights as long as they are not too heavy. Ask your provider how much you can lift. You don't need to join a gym or own particular equipment to stay active. You can walk in a safe environment or watch exercise DVDs at home. Alternatively, find methods to be active in your daily life, such as doing yard work or using the stairs instead of the elevator.

Is exercise safe for all pregnant women?
No. Some women are not able to exercise safely while pregnant. Your doctor can help you determine whether exercise is safe for you. The following conditions may make it dangerous to exercise while pregnant. Preterm labor, vaginal bleeding, or water bursts (also known as ruptured membranes).

Preterm labor occurs before 37 weeks of pregnancy. Preterm labor symptoms may include vaginal bleeding and a water break. Being pregnant with twins, triplets, or more (commonly known as multiples) and having additional risk factors for premature labor. If you are pregnant with multiples, ask your doctor if it is safe for you to exercise. Your provider may advise you not to engage in strenuous or high-impact activities, such as running. You might be able to practice low-impact activities like walking, prenatal yoga, or swimming.

Cervical insufficiency or cerclage. The cervix is the entryway to the uterus (womb), located at the top of the vagina. Cervical insufficiency (also known as incompetent cervix) occurs when your cervix opens (dilates) prematurely during pregnancy, typically without pain or contractions.

Cervical insufficiency can result in preterm delivery and miscarriage. If you have cervical insufficiency or a short cervix, your doctor may suggest cerclage. This is a stitch placed in your cervix to keep it closed and prevent your baby from being born prematurely.

A short cervix means that your cervix (also known as cervical length) is shorter than normal. Gestational hypertension, also known as preeclampsia. Gestational hypertension refers to elevated blood pressure during pregnancy. It begins after 20 weeks of pregnancy and ends after childbirth.

Placenta previa occurs after 26 weeks of pregnancy. This occurs when the placenta is very low in the uterus and completely or partially covers the cervix. The placenta develops in your uterus and provides the baby with food and oxygen via the umbilical cord. Placenta previa can lead to severe bleeding and other issues later in pregnancy. Severe anemia, or certain heart or lung diseases.

Anemia occurs when there aren't enough healthy red blood cells to deliver oxygen throughout your body. If you have a heart or lung issue, see your doctor about whether it is safe to exercise while pregnant.

What kind of activities are unsafe during pregnancy? When deciding on activities, exercise caution and consult with your clinician. During pregnancy, avoid doing: Any activity that involves jerky, bouncing movements that could cause you to tumble, such as horseback riding, downhill skiing, off-road cycling, gymnastics, or skateboarding. Any sport where you can be hit in the stomach, such as ice hockey, boxing, soccer, or basketball.

Any exercise that requires you to lie flat on your back (after the third month of pregnancy), such as sit-ups. When you lie on your back, your uterus presses on a vein that transports blood to your heart. Lying on your back can lower your blood pressure and reduce the flow of blood to your baby. Activities that can lead you to strike the water with significant force, such as water skiing, surfing, or diving. Skydive or scuba dive. Scuba diving can cause decompression sickness. This is when harmful gas bubbles grow throughout your baby's body.

Exercising at high altitude (above 6,000 feet), unless you reside at a high altitude. Altitude refers to the height of something above the earth. For example, if you're at a high elevation, you're presumably in the mountains.

Exercising at high elevations during pregnancy may reduce the amount of oxygen that reaches your baby. Activities that may raise your body temperature, such as Bikram yoga (also known as hot yoga) or exercising outside on hot, humid days. Bikram yoga takes place in a room with a temperature ranging from 95 to 100 degrees Fahrenheit. It is not safe for pregnant women since it can cause hyperthermia, a condition that occurs when the body's temperature rises too high.

Some studies suggest that spending too much time in a sauna or hot tub may raise your body temperature, increasing your chances of having a kid with birth abnormalities. To be safe, do not spend more than 15 minutes at a time in a sauna or 10 minutes in a hot tub.

Does pregnancy alter the way your body responds to exercise?

During pregnancy, your body undergoes various changes. When you're active, you can notice changes in Balance. You may find that you lose your balance more readily during pregnancy. Body temperature. Because your body temperature rises somewhat during pregnancy, you begin sweating earlier than usual. Breathing.

As your baby grows and your body changes, you require more oxygen. Your expanding belly puts pressure on your diaphragm, a muscle that aids in breathing. You may even have shortness of breath at times. Energy. Your body is working hard to care for your baby, so you may feel tired throughout pregnancy. Heart rate. During pregnancy, your heart pumps harder and faster to ensure that oxygen reaches your baby. Joints. During pregnancy, your body produces an increased level of several hormones. This can cause the tissues that support your joints to loosen. Try to avoid any motions that could strain or injure your joints. Hormones are substances produced by the body.

When should you quit exercising?

What are the warning indicators to look for when exercising? When you're exercising, drink plenty of water and pay attention to how your body feels. If you have any of the following signs or symptoms, stop your activity and notify your provider. Bleeding or leaking fluid from the vagina Chest discomfort, rapid heartbeat, or difficulty breathing Feeling dizzy or faint? Headache Muscle weakness, difficulty walking, soreness, or swelling in your lower legs. Pain or swelling in your lower legs may indicate deep vein thrombosis (DVT).

DVT occurs when a blood clot forms in a vein deep within the body, typically in the lower leg or thigh. If left untreated, it can result in major health complications and even death. Contractions are regular and painful. A contraction occurs when the muscles of your uterus tighten and then release.

Contractions help to push your baby out of your uterus. Your baby stops moving. This could be an indication of stillbirth (a baby dies in the womb after 20 weeks of pregnancy).

When can you resume exercising after giving birth?
Consult your healthcare physician to determine whether
it is safe for you to resume physical activity. If you had a
vaginal birth with no difficulties, you can normally begin
exercising a few days after giving birth or as soon as
you're ready. During vaginal birth, the uterus contracts to
help push your baby out of the birth canal.

If you had a c-section or experienced problems during
birth, you may need to wait longer to begin exercising
following birth. Your doctor can help you assess when
your body is ready to exercise. If you were active during
pregnancy, it will be easier to resume exercise once your
kid is delivered. Just start slow. If you have discomfort
or other issues while exercising, discontinue the activity
and consult your clinician.

CHAPTER 7

STRESS AND PREGNANCY

Being pregnant might cause you to experience a wide range of emotions, including anxiety and tension, but this is natural. Stress is a natural response to a significant change (such as pregnancy). Too much stress can be overwhelming and may result in health problems for both you and your kid.

What causes stress during pregnancy?
For some people, learning that they are pregnant can be a difficult event. You may feel out of control or as if you lack the resources to deal with what you will face. Stress can be caused by an unwanted pregnancy or by

becoming pregnant following previous traumatic experiences with pregnancy, birth, or motherhood, such as a miscarriage or the death of a baby. It can be hard to wait for the results of your antenatal tests and deal with the physical changes of pregnancy, especially if the pregnancy is challenging. Your home situation, such as being a single parent or teenager and wondering how you will manage, may stress you out.

Relationship issues, including family violence, may also have an effect. Pregnancy might present practical issues such as financial difficulties, relocating, and employment changes. Emotional pressures such as loss, prior worry, depression, or another mental disease, as well as drug and alcohol problems, can all contribute to increased stress during pregnancy. If more than one of the aforementioned events occurs simultaneously, you may experience additional stress.

How does stress affect my kid and me?
Chronic (ongoing) stress can hurt your health and well-being, causing headaches, difficulty sleeping, rapid breathing, and a racing pulse. Some people may also experience Obsessive thoughts. Worry or anxiety. Anger-related eating issues, including overeating, undereating, or consuming inappropriate foods.

Having difficulties relaxing or winding down Chronic stress may potentially cause issues for your baby. These can include effects on your unborn child's growth and the duration of your pregnancy (gestation). They can also increase the likelihood of problems with your baby's physical and mental development, as well as behavioral issues throughout childhood.

How can I lessen stress when pregnant?
During pregnancy, it is critical to care for both your emotional and physical health. When you are feeling good, pleased, and joyful, you can better manage stress. When you manage your stress, you and your kid are less likely to suffer significant consequences.

To relieve tension, try the following:

- Pay attention to the stress triggers and what happens when you're anxious.

- Try to calm down, rest, and avoid putting too much strain on yourself.

- Maintain a healthy, well-balanced diet to keep yourself and your baby healthy.

- Tell someone you trust about your concerns and how you are feeling.

- Physical activity and relaxation can also assist in relieving stress:

- Exercise regularly during pregnancy.

- Practice yoga, meditation, breathing techniques, or relaxation in class or with apps, videos, or podcasts.

- Engage in a favorite distracting activity, such as reading, watching television, or pursuing a hobby. Spend time with folks who make you feel relaxed. You don't have to cope on your own.

Try to ask for help when you need it and accept offers to assist you.

www.ingramcontent.com/pod-product-compliance
Lightning Source LLC
Chambersburg PA
CBHW051703250726

48653CB00007B/2817